Depression

Understanding the Black Dog

Depression

Understanding the Black Dog

Stephanie Sorrell

**PSYCHE
BOOKS**

Winchester, UK
Washington, USA

First published by Psyche Books, 2014
Psyche Books is an imprint of John Hunt Publishing Ltd., Laurel House, Station Approach,
Alresford, Hants, SO24 9JH, UK
office1@jhpbooks.net
www.johnhuntpublishing.com
www.psyche-books.com

For distributor details and how to order please visit the 'Ordering' section on our website.

Text copyright: Stephanie Sorrell 2013

ISBN: 978 1 78279 165 2

A CIP catalogue record for this book is available from the British Library.

Design: Lee Nash

Printed and bound by CPI Group (UK) Ltd, Croydon, CR0 4YY

We operate a distinctive and ethical publishing philosophy in all
areas of our business, from our global network of authors to
production and worldwide distribution.

CONTENTS

Acknowledgements

For my publisher, Maria Barry of *Psyche Books*, for seeing the potential in this work and especially for her enduring patience in waiting for the finished manuscript to materialize!

Special commendations to Hanne Jahr, my best friend, for her patience and critical proofreading skills. And most of all, for suggesting I wrote this book in the first place.

Not least of all, to John Hunt's energy and long internship to keep all these wonderful imprints going.

Author's Previous Publications

The River that Knows the Way: an anthology of wisdom and beauty
The Hamblin Trust, 1997

Trusting the Process
The Hamblin Trust, 2000

Depression as a Spiritual Journey
John Hunt Publishing, 2009

Nature as Mirror, an ecology of body, mind and soul
John Hunt Publishing, 2001

Psychosynthesis (Made Easy series)
O-books, 2011

The Therapist's Cat
Soul Rocks, 2012

Astral Projection and overcoming the fear of death (Made Easy series)
Sixth Books, 2012

Self Unbandaged (poetry of the soul)
Chipmunka publishing, 2013

Introduction

Depression is a direct result of our attempts to be happy all the time.
Mary Rose

In order to fully understand what the Black Dog is, it is important to look at the polar opposite of depression which, loosely defined, is a sense of well-being, purpose and meaning. This can be a sense of 'feeling at home with ourselves' in the world. Our happiness may be a natural state of being derived from involving ourselves in a goal or work we enjoy, family and relationships or both. Happiness is where purpose, meaning and value are engaged. As primarily social beings, it is vital to experience a sense of belonging in our environment, manifesting through family, work, colleagues and friends and, if we are lucky — all three.

On the premise of this, the recipe for happiness appears to be quite straightforward. Purpose is unique to us all. For some, it may be taking pride in a garden, working with the seasons, planting seeds or bedding plants into a border. The satisfaction or reward in this is in witnessing the cycle of shoots emerging through the soil, to the blossoming, ripening of fruit or bud into blossom. Others may derive satisfaction from baking cakes, making bread or jam, or preparing for the next social event, a dinner party or family get-together. Still others may anticipate a longed-for holiday; going on a trek across the Himalayas or merely a visit to a warmer climate. If our time at work is mundane, tedious or stressful our inner sense of well-being may be rooted in the company of supportive friends, pets, grand-children or an engaging hobby like scuba diving or getting involved in one of the many conservation projects worldwide.

On a more attainable and mundane level, listening to music, reading a book or watching a video may suffice. More creative people may take time to express themselves by writing a book, painting a picture or designing a poster. Hard work and being one pointed is a way of channeling frustration and depression in a more creative direction as illustrated in chapter 2. When there is difficulty and conflict, there is a longing for meaning, purpose and value. This can manifest on a spiritual level where depth and vision are sought as demonstrated in chapter 3.

Intrinsically, like the layers of an onion, we consist of complementary levels of expression and need. These levels of being as physician and homeopathic practitioner, Mabel Agahdiu lists in her excellent book, *Soul Matters, the spiritual dimension in Healthcare*, consist of five levels of manifestation:

Cultural
Spiritual
Physical
Mental
Psychological

For each individual, these levels of identification and expression vary in significance and value according to personal and cultural experience. For example, a predominately somatic person is someone who identifies strongly with their physical world through their senses and body. They may work out regularly at the gym, go running or cycling regularly each week. If this focus becomes eclipsed by a physical injury which needs a long process of rehabilitation, their focus may undergo a total catharsis in outlook. Through time and frustration, value and identification may shift to a psychological awareness through a need to process his experience and sense of loss. Crises in any shape or form, shatters ones current values and erodes the framework of what was once held to be important. For many people who become depressed and, in an effort to find guidance and meaning, will begin to identify with the spiritual component of their life.

Belonging to a spiritual community in a time of crisis confers a much needed social network. Not only that, but it addresses psychological needs of belonging and cohesion. In the face of disaster and loss, spiritual value is often sought as shown in chapter 9.

As youngsters, our social network plays a vital role in our sense of belonging in the world. If we lack this amongst our peers, we become depressed and isolated. Social networks not only define who we are, but they engage us with the needs of others. In the language of group dynamics, the 'whole' is always stronger than the 'parts'. Because of our inherent need to fit into a group identity, there is a tendency in the young to sacrifice all sense of moral responsibility.

But, supposing we don't fit into the social framework around us? We can feel ostracized and disconnected, making us vulnerable to losing our ground and sometimes our moral compass as we struggle to fit into any social network in order to belong. In short, belonging to a social network can override all moral and societal injunctions in the young troubled person. I do believe that unidentified depression underlies a lot of crime in young people, especially males, which makes early diagnosis so important. The finalizing chapter, *The Value of Depression*, opens up a relatively unexplored or recognized byproduct of the Black Dog—that it might have value in the form of creativity. Although I have not covered the creative process, I have described this at great length in my previous book, *Depression as a Spiritual Journey*. It is from this work that I have included an abridged copy of the value of medication to address deep and unremitting depression. This works very effectively on a therapeutic level. Unlike psychiatric medications of the past, the medications of today are far less sedating than the old ones; not only that, they are designed to work specifically on particular neurotrans-mitters. After being antagonistic towards the invasion of a 'chemical cosh' for some time, I have learned through experience that medication is just as important in some cases, as medical intervention in the form of warfarin and beta-blockers are for the ailing heart. Both conditions are potentially life threatening.

Chapter 1

Is Depression Really that Serious?

Yes!

300 million Americans are depressed at any given time! 75,000 lives are lost through depression globally each year. Furthermore, suicide is the leading course of death in the male population of 15-24-year-olds.

That *is* serious!

Statistics reveal depression is increasing and that it is, currently, the third biggest cause of death behind heart disease and stroke. It is estimated that by 2030 it will move up to second place. One million people are desperate enough to commit suicide each year. Although older men dominate the statistics for taking their own lives, younger people, especially males, overcome by social and financial expectations are opting out too. The impossible expectations to be rich and successful channeled endlessly through the media does little to help.

But these are not the only reasons.

Depression is a 'dis-ease' which runs like bedrock through every strata of society, from rich to poor, from the intellectual to the person with learning difficulties. Depression is not class conscious. It infiltrates all sectors of our modern world. Although this reads like a missive of hopelessness and failure, in all honesty, depression cannot be fully addressed or understood until the facts are known. This work is all about understanding the Black Dog, getting to know it, familiarizing ourselves with its behavior, rather than benchmarking it as something to be fought or bludgeoned senseless. Later, I want to explore the *value* of it and how this can be utilized creatively rather than working against us.

If the majority of people pay homage to the mindset that

depression has no underlying value and therefore is a total waste of time, not to mention resources, depression is never going to go away. Italian psychiatrist, Roberto Assagioli, the founder of Psychosynthesis Psychology's well-known maxim was, 'That which is denied rules'. I have found this denial to be prevalent in diverse social groups, as well as impacting on every level of society. Climate change denial has been paramount for some time, especially where the cost of implementing defensive measures is, as Lord Stern, British Environment Adviser, asserts, ' ranks very low in the political agenda.' We deny climate change at our own peril. I am writing this in the midst of the River Thames, among other rivers, breaking their flood defenses. The natural environment, like depression, is very much in the driving seat.

What isn't addressed and brought to the surface festers and grows in power until, like a ripe boil, it explodes onto the surface. There is the mistaken belief that what isn't focused on, somehow goes away. Hunger doesn't go away, however much we ignore it. Hunger and starvation, like depression, run like a fault line throughout the world. The more we ignore it, the bigger it becomes, eroding the boundaries of our collective and individual conscience. Although, it is tempting to repress what we are uncomfortable with in the unconscious, that which is repressed returns to haunt its oppressor whether it be the chemicals we bury in the earth, or uncomfortable memories emerging from the battleground of war.

In the next chapter, I want to explore the various levels which depression manifests on. These in short, range from *mild*, *moderate* to *major* depression. The information here can be used as a barometer to measure the level of intensity suffering manifests on, along with the therapeutic intervention needed to address each level.

Chapter 2

The Levels of Depression

The major error we make in understanding depression is in lumping all types of depression under one fuzzy heading. For this reason, delineating the levels on which depression manifests is absolutely key to our understanding. Therapeutic intervention of any kind can only work if it meets the level of need. Rather than depression forming a large amorphous mass which engulfs the population at random, it becomes defined and distinctly tangible. Basically, we are afraid of what we cannot understand, define or fix. In this light, our current level of fear and general ignorance around depression spirals out of control, making us defensive and judgmental.

Relegated to near plague status, any understanding which may be available, the depressed person stands accused in the dock and found guilty of bringing it upon themselves. What a loaded message! But—I am not exaggerating. Although our understanding is growing, psychological and social progress is slow to keep up with the fast emerging evidence that the majority of depression is rooted in the genes and physical body. Rather than a 'dis-ease' brought upon ourselves through faulty thinking. This does not mean that we should do nothing to help ourselves or feel doomed by the label. Rather, we can stop blaming ourselves for having depression and find a way of working *with* it rather than against it through medical and psychological intervention. Today, there are many forms of therapeutic intervention available, not all of them costing a fortune. There are many self-help groups available, particularly in the West.

Yet—on the heels of this, I have to say that *reactive depression* falls into a different category altogether and can be addressed with Cognitive Behavior Therapy (CBT). Reactive depression has a definite cause and by backtracking to a defining event or series of events can be helpful in bringing conscious awareness to the matter. Reactive depression affects us all to a greater or lesser extent and is nothing to be ashamed of. Once realized, steps can be taken to break the destructive cycle. And remember, no experience, however galling, is without value. Psychotherapists can take years to train and learn about the various levels mental imbalances can rest on. Some of the best therapists have been through 'hell' themselves. Understanding their own personal traumas in an adult way, rather than regressing into a 'wounded child' status, can create the proving ground for a first-class psychotherapist or counselor.

Who can fail to be moved by the injury or death of a close relative or friend? Or the crumbling of a close relationship, or the loss of a job? Indeed, if we have the tendency, we can sink into a deep unremitting depression after any life trauma. However, in vulnerable individuals who may not have the skills or self-awareness to process their own disappointments, mild and moderate depression can jackknife into major depression.

If CBT were part of the mandatory curriculum in schools, this would equip young people with the tools to cope with adversity in their everyday life. Instead, trying to emulate the plethora of contestants on the endless talent shows creates an impossible dream which, for many, sets one up for huge disappointment when success and fame doesn't happen.

When the British government designated a plan in the 1990s to train up 10,000 health professionals in CBT, the level of depression they aimed to address was mild to moderate depression. CBT works on the premise that we have the ability to change our outlook by following a simple program. For example, an elderly client may find themselves becoming depressed about the state of her carpet with all the family walking in and out spilling crumbs and drinks onto the floor. A CBT practitioner would, perhaps, *reframe* the problem by remarking on the amount of people who want to visit the client each day. Perhaps, they would suggest that human companionship can be more important than a few crumbs on the carpet.

Basically, the intention is good. Why waste time trawling the tricky and not always helpful minefield of medication for a condition that will respond well to cognitive strategies, enabling the client to manage and reform their way of thinking? In this sense, the mildly depressed person can gain some personal autonomy through understanding their thought patterns. With practice, and taking into account the neuro-plasticity of the brain, the client can consciously create new pathways of thinking which bypass the destructive censoring of the less conscious brain.

However...

Approaching major depression with similar cognitive exercises alone will rarely succeed — simply because the individual's ability to even think or put one foot in front of the other is severely compromised by their medical condition. In order to benefit from CBT one needs to have a brain and body that is working. However positive your intentions, in major depression you cannot *think* your way out of this because, basically, the neural chemistry is malfunctioning. Sadly, many people with major depression feel they have failed if they haven't the will or cognitive pliability to follow the program laid out for them. Their sense of failure and frustration can be so overwhelming that it further exacerbates the depression rather than alleviating the pain of it. But if medication is stabilizing the depression, the severely depressed person may be able to process CBT and gain some value from it.

Depression is often grouped under three headings:

Mild
Moderate
Major

Mild Depression

Everyone at some time feels depressed which can be due to variations in the weather, exam results, hormonal fluctuations, social and work pressures or the disappointment of having something that was long anticipated, canceled. Every level of society, young and old, are familiar with mild depression. Animals can suffer depression too if they are ill-treated or lose an important family member. Mild depression can be alleviated by tackling a long pending project such as decorating a room or clearing the attic. Although this, in psychological terms, is known as *displacement therapy*, it is a very effective way of managing stress and working with disappointment and frustration. These long pending tasks can sap our energy and give rise to low level depression. After completing one of these 'back boiler' tasks, it is surprising how much lighter we feel. Unfinished business does, over time, sap our energy which can be the precursor to depression.

As time passes, we develop various coping strategies to address life's disappointments. If the weather gets us down in the form of endless rain, dark winters or the cloying humidity of a heat wave, we can usually meet the inconvenience creatively, by doing something more suitable or simply just letting it all go—if we can. If we are financially able, a holiday abroad to a different climate can diffuse a sense of being stuck. Also, exercise such as jogging or cycling is validated by most healthcare professionals as exercise releases the 'feel good' endorphins in the brain.

There is fluidity with mild depression which makes change more accessible.

But...

The fundamental problem here is this: many people who have experienced mild depression will only have awareness at this level and believe that *all* depression is mild – yet grossly blown out of proportion by those who cannot take a few knocks. The fallout from a loss or disappointment is often classified as *reactive depression* which can nosedive into moderate and major depression. Yet, within each failure and loss lies an opportunity. Since adversity is an integral part of life and is not always connected with what we are doing wrong or right—it just is—we can adapt to this and grow. Instead of having a gut reaction to a problem or obstacle, we can ask ourselves: 'What is the opportunity in this?'

Remember, nothing is wrong with depression itself or adversity. In fact, quite the opposite, it can teach us empathy and understanding together with the ability to help and enable others to find value in their pain. It is sad that the least understood conditions in life have a very strong 'blame culture'. Depression 'just is'. Many animals suffer from it through loss of habitat, captivity and cruelty. As human beings we adapt and grow but have the added bonus of managing our mood by discovering what works for us, individually.

Not unlike other pathological conditions, even mild depression can be hereditary, not necessarily because it reproduces through learned behavior, but simply because there are genetic markers in the family matrix which predispose us to particular conditions such as arthritis and eczema or cardiac problems in later life. These markers need not be negative, they can be positive too, in the form of creativity, a 'head' for figures or a natural leaning towards gymnastics or athletics. Even a strong will can be passed on genetically!

Symptoms of Mild Depression

Like most depression, there is a tendency to feel worse in the morning
Anxiety
A sense of impending doom
Fluctuations in appetite and sleep patterns
Restlessness along with a need to 'get away' or have a change
Retail therapy
Moving the furniture around in the house

Feelings of low self-worth
Irritability
Guilt
Emotional instability
Self-criticism
Fluctuations between social isolation and excessive socialization
Mood swings
Resorting to alcohol in order to dull the sense of isolation

Moderate to Major Depression

It is more than likely that anyone suffering from moderate to major depression is displaying a hereditary condition from their family of origin. This doesn't mean that if one of your parents or your grandmother suffered from depression, that you will. It just increases the statistics. Most diagnosed cases of depression fall under this category. A large proportion of people here may find their moods dipping and soaring in correspondence to the changing seasons as in Seasonal Affective Disorder (SAD). During the summer months, depression will usually lift and possibly polarize to intense feelings of well-being. This type of depressive episode manifests cyclically throughout one's life. Although Bipolar Disorder can fall into this category, I open this out more extensively in the next chapter to avoid any confusion.

Post-natal depression is another type of depression which also falls under this category and can be both debilitating and unexpected, undermining one's ability to reach out for help or even function. Aside from this, there are societal injunctions about being a 'bad mum', further exacerbating an endless tide of guilt around not being able to cope.

Symptoms

Like all depression, symptoms are worse in the morning, tending to ease off as the day progresses.

Sleeplessness
Loss of appetite
Low self-esteem
Self-criticism
A need to isolate oneself from others
Reduced,or fluctuations in sex drive
Inability to concentrate
Forgetfulness
Lethargy in movement and speech, along with an overall sense of
    being slowed down, or 'driving with the brakes on'
Suicidal thoughts which may require intervention through hospital-
    ization and medication
Self-harming

There are many different ways of managing and alleviating the discomfort of depression, but it is important to address the depression at the level it manifests on or else we can do much more harm than good. For example, for someone who is suicidal and is self-harming, the intervention of CBT or psychoanalyses at this critical and volatile point is likely to do more harm than good.

Certainly, when I was at my lowest, I had to give up weekly psychotherapy, which was part of the training module for my degree. This was because my thinking had slowed down to such a degree, that there was *no way* I could have strung more than one thought together, let alone verbalized it. Most of the time, I felt like one of those houseflies caught in the gluey film of sticky flypaper where everything was blurred, painful and indistinct. What I needed was something I had fought against in my earlier years, to my detriment. This was the *right* medication that could hold me together until I was well enough again. Although I was barely able to walk, let alone speak, I had a strong enough 'observing self' to understand what was happening to me. I knew I was very ill and needed a safe place to be until the medication began to work. During deep and unremitting depression, before you reach that state of numbness, the feelings become so strong that cognitive thought doesn't get a look in – however hard you try.

I have learned from Psychiatrist, Tim Cantopher, the reason why this is so in his insightful book, *Depressive Illness, the Curse of the Strong*. He describes how the limbic system, or old mammalian brain, came into being 300 million years ago when the first mammals walked the earth. The mammalian brain, among other things, controls appetite, sleep-wake cycles and hormones which are all affected in major depression. The limbic system, also known as the emotional brain, will always override the prefrontal cortex which is a relative newcomer to the brain network. It is the prefrontal cortex which looks out for our safety by keeping us tethered to instincts and hunches. When we get that bolt of lightning which galvanizes us into instinctive reactions, that is the reptilian brain or the cerebellum, which is our hind brain. Although ancient, it is vital to our survival. Basically the reptilian brain is instinctive, the mammalian brain emotive and the prefrontal lobes are responsible for our thinking.

Sadly, particularly in men, there is a lot of shame attached to depression and becomes the reason why suicide is, too often, the chosen method of intervention in the male population. Shame, in itself, is one of the most debilitating and corrosive of emotions.

In Japan, where the culture of shame and stigmatism towards depression is endemic, suicide is high. According to the *Japan Times* one in five of the population is depressed at any given period. Here, particularly, suicide is high among the male population. *Japan Times* writer, Roger Pulvas, believes that the only hope for dispersion of this stigmatism is if enough high profile people, such as movie stars and pop singers admit to suffering from depression. Although this is happening with more and more frequency amongst the female population, men are still dragging their heels because they think mental health problems are a form of weakness.

This is very unfortunate because something that punches a hole through the close network of family and friends should not have to suffer shame on top of the loss of life and connection. It is important that continued research and news coverage is widely circulated to break this cycle of shame.

Yet, the high profile and rising incidence of cardiac disease is believed to be intimately connected with depression, simply because depression affects the clotting factor in blood platelets, As psychiatrist, Peter Kramer writes:

Depression is not merely a brain disease. It is a neurologic, hematologic and cardiovascular disease. Over-activation of stress pathways causes a liability to clots and arrhythmias. These factors alone predispose heart attacks, silent strokes, disturbed mood and sudden death.

Additionally, he describes how serotonin-based antidepressants act on blood clotting and heart rhythm. This factor alone should be enough to turn the tide of ambivalence towards depression.

Chapter 3

Bipolar Disorder

The light that burns twice as brightly, burns half as long.
Blade Runner (SF film)

Bipolar Disorder is usually an inherited condition, working its way through the family matrix from generation to generation. Although there are episodes of euphoria, particularly in Bipolar 1, this can be accompanied by unrelenting troughs of depression, anxiety and psychosis which can extend into weeks or months.

Yet—on this dizzying rollercoaster of mood swings, much of our literary and artistic insights have been produced. There is ample evidence of this emerging through the lives of many creative people throughout history; people such as Virginia Woolf, John Keats, Thomas Chatterton, Sylvia Plath, Oscar Wilde, John Ruskin, Gerard Manley Hopkins and Elizabeth Barrett Browning. On a more contemporary level, creative individuals have emerged through the media in the form of comedian Stephen Fry, singer Sinead O'Connor, Catherine Zeta Jones and Kurt Cobain. More recently, people with Bipolar 1 have been able to manage their mood swings with a mixture of mood stabilizers, lithium and antidepressants which are now more tailored to address explicit conditions.

Symptoms of Bipolar 1 (Mania)

Restlessness/agitation
Excitement/euphoria
Increased energy
Racing thoughts/lots of ideas
A need for very little sleep

Loss of appetite through excessive excitement
Feelings of omnipotence ·
Narcissistic thoughts/delusions of grandeur
Increased sexual activity
Impulsive and compulsive buying
Depression and suicidal thoughts
Hallucinations

Due to severe mood swings, individuals suffering from bipolar 1 invariably have a checkered working career. Long and sustained periods of being able to work consistently in the outside world are eclipsed by paranoid episodes, manic activity which makes work impossible to sustain. A job or career which offers the ability to work on an 'ad hoc' basis can be the only option. Many people with bipolar 1 work for themselves because of their mood fluctuations and variable work output. It takes a very sympathetic employer in today's economic climate, to back or put their weight behind an unreliable 'horse' even though performance levels can be outstanding at times. As the bipolar personality seems to favor a highly creative temperament, many artists, writers, performers, actors and musicians are able to work for themselves.

I have a number of bipolar friends who are musicians and several who work as artists. Whether they would have leaned towards creativity if they were not bipolar is difficult to assess. But creativity is a very powerful and constructive way of managing a debilitating condition.

American Psychiatrist, Kay Redfield Jamison who suffers from bipolar 1 herself has written some of the most definitive works on bipolar disorder. Her insight both as a sufferer and practitioner in the field of psychiatric medicine are, historically, some of the most informative on this condition. In her iconic work, *Touched with Fire,* Jamison writes compellingly about her bipolar disorder and how it has hounded many creative individuals throughout history.

Of course, the ability to function in the world is dependent on the efficacy of medication together with the severity of the condition and accessibility to the right psychiatrist.

Because the 'highs' associated with bipolar 1 are so dizzyingly ebullient, there is a sense of the transpersonal. At this point, the bipolar person can feel invincible as their thinking becomes conflated with delusions of grandeur and a sense of omnipotence. On one level, the person is both manic and having a spiritual experience which, later, can be an ongoing struggle to integrate in the psyche. I explore this further in my book, *Depression as a Spiritual Journey*. Here, the recipient of the released energy so identifies with their omnipotence that they can even believe they *are* God as uncontrollable, narcissistic feelings flood the consciousness. The individual, unable to process this energy psychologically, may carry out acts which endanger his life; leaping across railway tracks, jumping from buildings, with detrimental results. On one level, they are having a profound spiritual experience and, on another, they appear manic, deranged, out of themselves. In bipolar 1, although there are lows and periods of depression, they are rarely as severe and life-threatening as that experienced in bipolar 2.

Bipolar 2

Bipolar 2 can be defined as cyclical mood swings which never quite reach full-blown mania. Often it is regarded as less serious than Bipolar 1 because the highs are not so extreme. Like bipolar 1, there is often a tendency to grandiosity and lucid fast flowing thoughts. But this is not always the case, as there is a greater incidence of plummeting into 'suicidal depths' for long and protracted periods. Internment in desperate moods and thoughts can have a detrimental effect on the individual concerned, but also his close relatives and friends. In some cases, as depressive conditions don't age particularly well, suicidal thoughts may be acted out more than once in a lifetime.

Fortunately, bipolar 2 usually responds well to medication. Thanks to a psychotherapist I was seeing as a mandatory component of my degree, I took her advice in getting my medication sorted out early on in the therapy— as this would stabilize the mood swings and suicidal feelings which plagued me. Although there are some bodies of thought who still believe medication antagonizes the efficacy of therapy, this seems to be changing. The two can complement each other very effectively. Treating depression is rarely an either/or program, but can benefit from several approaches simultaneously. I have found medication to work very well with counseling in the past. In this sense, medication stabilizes the mood as a prerequisite to effective counseling. This combination of therapies plays out effectively in treating physiological functions, where muscular spasms can benefit from exercise as well as the medication to address the spasms.

Symptoms

Seasonal changes in mood, particularly in the spring and fall
Deep unremitting depression in the spring, accompanied by euphoria in the late summer
A tendency to 'cycle' down low in the fall
Feelings of well-being, enthusiasm and joy
Fluctuations in energy and mood
Creative ideas and insights
Clear, lucid thoughts
Variations in sleep patterns
Extended periods of depression, agitation and anxiety
Inertia, exhaustion, desperation
Restlessness, with a need to get away/move to a different location (in an effort to escape oneself!)

Treatment

For clinical depression a psychotherapist is not always the first choice of intervention for addressing this issue. This is because the person in the grip of clinical depression is not always thinking clearly or has the ability to process any plan of action. Psychotherapy links mood disorders to personal history which might be true in some cases, but certainly not in major depression. In fact, any criticism, whether intentional or not, may be enough to push someone with clinical depression over a very dangerous edge. For anyone who is not sure of the difference between a counseling or psychotherapeutic approach, I will make a distinction between the two. Basically, a counselor deals with the presenting problem and works to find a way for the client to manage it by applying a different perspective. Each level of therapeutic intervention has value, but certainly there needs to be some understanding of this before a decision is made.

Counseling is usually the first choice, as this is less invasive, more life-affirming and cognitively suitable for when in the vice-like grip of deep depression. Skills are needed here to work with the client's mood and learn to accept the 'discomfort' in a supportive non-judgmental way. Patience and the ability to sit in the silence with the client for long periods is very therapeutic, once the client has bypassed the initial discomfort. Yet... this may be all the depressed person needs; an unquestioning acceptance from another human being. It is also in this medium of silence that emotions, memories and feelings have the opportunity to emerge.

There are many forms of counseling and psychotherapy available. For example, Freudian psychoanalysis is very different from Cognitive Behavior Therapy (CBT) or Humanistic counseling. If a spiritual dimension is sought then Jungian therapy can work very well with its symbolic language. Psychosynthesis counseling combines many different approaches and brings them all under a spiritual wing, principally referred to as the 'Self'. Additionally, it includes the element of 'soul' in the therapy. Really, all psychologies should embrace this – since 'psyche' in translation, means 'soul'! The Jungian template includes dream-work which is another, less invasive, way for the client to integrate his mind and emotions. I can strongly recommend psychosynthesis counseling as a therapy because it works to integrate the body, mind and soul.

Chapter 4

How we are Affected by the Weather

We should never underestimate the power of seasonal fluctuations to affect the mood and well-being of individuals and groups of people.

Most people are affected by seasonal fluctuations in weather – from the dark oppressive winters to the lengthening days. Group and individual performance is woven through these seasonal and diurnal variations. On a clear, bright day, few people remain unaffected by the presence of sunshine. Living in the UK, where the winter months can be long, dark, wet and oppressive, most people change in the presence of sunshine and become more outgoing. People I haven't seen for weeks appear from some invisible amphitheatre and smile at each other in a way that they don't when it is dark and oppressive.

Biologically, our inner climate has been intimately connected to nature's cycles. It is for this reason that, globally, there is surprising leniency and mitigating factors when the weather can be held to ransom instead. Crimes that are committed in the form of road accidents and temper-fueled incidents when the Mistral blows in Southern France, are treated in a less punitive way. These are known locally as 'witch winds', and are believed to contain an abundance of positive ions which affect both mind and body in an adverse way. Not surprisingly, when these ill winds blow, there are more hospital admissions with cardiac, respiratory and psychiatric problems than in more temperate conditions.

In contrast, when 'negative ions' are released in the atmosphere after a rainstorm, around running water or by the sea, they can induce a calming, sometimes mildly euphoric effect on the mind and body. We only have to watch children in the school playground when fall or spring winds blow. Their excitement and euphoria is tangible. Farm animals, too, become playful and skittish as do domestic creatures. Interestingly enough, negative ions speed up the rate in which serotonin is oxidized in the blood stream which, in this context, has an important bearing on mood and well-being.

Similarly, stormy, overcast weather affects many people in a negative way and this is usually due to the absence of light which stimulates the pineal gland. This small pea-shaped structure in the mid brain produces light-sensitive cells which increase the production of melatonin in the body enabling us to relax. Natural daylight is vital to our sense of well-being as serotonin, that feel-good factor, production increases. It is good to be aware of this, particularly in the winter months, especially when wearing sunglasses which block this chemical exchange. Additionally, both meditation and sleep complement the production of melatonin.

Norman Rosenthal, a South African psychiatrist, validated the authenticity of Seasonal Depression in the 1980s. He believed that the changing seasons affected many people in an adverse way, destabilizing emotional and psychological equilibrium. Furthermore, he noticed that the seasons affected people with major depression, especially; sometimes sending those affected into an episode of suicidal depression or out-of-control euphoria. We can be grateful for his pioneering work in promoting the importance of 'light' treatment for seasonal depression. Among other benefits of light therapy is the therapeutic effect on eczema, psoriasis and jaundice. Similarly, French Philosopher and mathematician, Descartes, referred to the pineal gland as the 'seat of the soul' which he describes in his own words:

Playing a decisive role in bodily functions, monitoring the work of the glands and organs, and regulating hormone production. It also controls over-stimulation of the sympathetic nerves to lower blood pressure and slow the heart rate, thus reducing the impact on the heart. It alleviates mental stress, improves sleep, adjusts the body's biological clock, relieves jet lag, strengthens immunity, increases the body's resistance to germs and viruses, and prevents cancer and senile dementia.

In the next chapter we will explore one of depression's overriding symptoms which undermines every level of communication including the social, physical, cognitive and spiritual.

Chapter 5

Disconnection

For most people, one of the defining characteristics of depression is a sense of disconnection with the world around them. Because of this, there is a desire to withdraw from social networks at a time when they are most *needed*. It is as if the world is going on around the depressed person, but they cannot be a part of it because an invisible screen stands in the way. Depression seems to confine one to a crystallized state where body and mind lack any inherent sense of cohesion. Even the most rudimentary skills, such as making a telephone call, appear to be beyond one's capability. Preparing and cooking a meal seems so remote from our internal experience that it becomes an insurmountable feat.

It is not uncommon for depressed people to lose their appetite or graze endlessly on calorie-laden food which offers very little nourishment. In short, body and mind are not in communication with each other because they lack an inherent sense of connectivity. The depressed person's world not only slows down—but regresses to a basic survival level of barely sleeping, eating and barely functioning. It is not a matter of being apathetic or lazy; it is simply due to the 'the hard disk of the brain become jammed'.

Sleep is something tantalizingly out of reach for the severely depressed person. When sleep does descend, even for a few minutes, they jerk, heart racing with anxiety, only to find that the rest of the night stretches out ahead in a tortured canvas of wakefulness, dread, anxiety and anguish. Self-punishing thoughts gnaw into the darkness of the long wakeful night. Night and day seem to be ominously conflated with little respite available. Appetite is so diminished that even the thought of preparing a meal fills one with nausea. Natural hunger seems to have vacated the sufferer completely. Normally, when the depressed person is at work, they relish the idea of days stretching ahead in the form of a holiday or break. But now, hounded by self-critical thoughts, one's only desire is to escape all the mental anguish. At this stage, the Black Dog is rampant, shredding away at any thoughts which may offer even the remotest salve to a mind tortured out of control. Although needing help, it seems impossible to actualize this because the idea of picking up the telephone and talking to a receptionist seems an impossible task. The person in the grip of the Black Dog can no more 'pull him/herself together'–whatever that is—than life can continue running smoothly in the midst of a hurricane or tornado.

Again, it is important to remind ourselves that moderate to major depression is a serious illness. Disconnection is exactly what it says – an inability to connect to different parts of our brain and body. Since the precursors of connectivity are serotonin-fueled neurotransmitters, the magical chemical which connects thoughts together, it surely can be no surprise that our ability to function is severely impaired. Like an aging computer, we are dysfunctional.

The good news is that there is plenty of help available. But the greatest hurdle is going to the doctor and seeking advice. It is tragic that any move to help ourselves seems to be ridden with conflict as societal injunctions rush in to deflect us from our quest in the form of guilt, fear and shame.

After all, the Black Dog's identity and presence is *dependent* on our neurotransmitters not working, on our feeling isolated and disconnected. Be aware of this, as you try to heal yourself or a friend or relative. Consciousness and understanding of yourself, especially if it affects your thoughts and behavior, always bring up conflict and fear. Because *change is dangerous!* No human or non-human animal likes a change in routine, even if our health depends on it.

As we mature in outlook and, this may have very little to do with physical years, we develop the ability to see and discern the *value* of challenging situations in our life. In a sense, they define us and make us who we are. Later, I want to focus on the value and gifts that can be harnessed from Black Dog. This challenges the present mindset that depression has no purpose or meaning.

Chapter 6

Neurotransmitters and Exercise

The Black Dog isn't very keen on exercise. Remember to take him for a walk each day. He might decide to go off on his own and leave you alone for a while.

Although the work of neurotransmitters is very much in the foreground when addressing depression, and we might already be aware that they have something to do with mental dexterity and our ability to function properly, it is useful to be reminded of what they do more in depth.

Basically neurotransmitters are the chemicals which relay information backwards and forwards from our brain to the body. They do this by activating signals between nerve cells, also known as neurons. Most of the time, they work efficiently in the background and we are not conscious of them until something goes wrong. Aside from communicating with the major organs of the body – signaling the lungs to breathe, the heart to beat, the kidneys to process its fluids, they can affect mood and appetite. One of these neurotransmitters is serotonin which, because it is an inhibitory transmitter, calms the nervous system when it is over-stressed. It also affects body weight, appetite and the sleep cycle. If there is a deficiency in serotonin, due to excitatory transmitters or stimulants like coffee and certain kinds of recreational drugs which drain the serotonin supply, mood, sleep and general well-being are adversely effected. Dopamine, another important neurotransmitter, give us a sense of well-being and happiness when we have achieved something, like a good painting, passing an exam or tackling an activity that we have put off for too long. Because dopamine is a feel-good chemical, there is always the danger of addiction. The recreational game industry knows this and creates computer games which target the pleasure center for people, causing them to *want* more, in the way of food, or the latest product. Many addictive drugs like cocaine and LSD enhance dopamine levels. Because dopamine is connected to physical exercise, its heightened levels, along with the increase of serotonin, can give rise to a 'runner's high'. That's why many of us feel so good after exercise, and can become addicted to it. Chicago Science editor, Steven Connor, cites a study involving the effect of exercise on 120 people aged between 60-80 with quite astonishing results. The study revealed that just by walking briskly 30-40 minutes a day, three times a week was all that it took to 're-grow the structures of the brain linked to cognitive decline.' Not only that, brain scans taken before and after the year-long study revealed that the prefrontal cortex and the hippocampus grew in volume. This was compared with another group just doing stretching exercises whose brains continued to shrink. In short, regular exercise sustains the neuro-plasticity of the brain. Furthermore, six months of exercise can increase the size of the hippocampus which is involved with memory and learning, the area that the aging process effects the most. A case study revealed that a man diagnosed with early Alzheimer's disease was, when out running, able to engage in conversation and feel more connected to the world.

A large sector of the advertising industry thrives on targeting three activities which feed into the reward center of the brain, the part involved in dopamine production. These are *food, sex and novelty.* It is common knowledge that low levels of dopamine are symptomatic of Parkinson's disease which compromises speech, movement and mood, leaving the person trapped inside a rigid or shaking body. This is made evident in the iconic film, *Awakenings,* based on the book by the neurologist, Oliver Sacks. Although the neurotransmitters work unconsciously in the background, it is worth keeping a diary of mood cycles in connection with exercise and certain types of food. Serotonin-rich foods include almonds, sunflower seeds, fish oil and flax oil. Since exercise increases tryptophan which is a precursor of serotonin, this is an integral part of an everyday working program. Even walking briskly 30 minutes each day can be enough to boost the mood, if only to harness enough light in the pineal gland. In contrast with artificial lighting in buildings, homes and hospitals which all block the natural serotonin production in the brain, even a dull day can have a positive effect on mood. There is enough light or Lux even on a dull day to lift serotonin levels in the brain.

Chapter 7

The Role of Medication

The journey from being medication free to taking medication for the clinically depressed is one riddled with apprehension, resistance, ambivalence and desperation. The idea that depressed or anxious people mindlessly pop pills without foresight or consideration for the long-term implications is a complete myth. Taking medication is not only a loss of personal autonomy and self-esteem, but also an admission that one has a genuine medical condition which warrants treatment. Powerful feelings which may have closed the door to treatment before are shattered. In their place, there are often feelings of intense shame and failure that one is unable to cope any more.

The movement from non-medication to medication is a non-linear process. It is based on escalating, progressively more debilitating episodes of depression to periods of relative normality. This cycle of normality can last more than six or twelve months, even longer, but always seems to reappear in moments of vulnerability.

When a person has a sudden relapse, too often this is because the individual has come off their medication too quickly or cut down to a dangerously low level which can only add fuel to another episode. Within this process there may be visits to the GP with an assortment of vague, seemingly unrelated symptoms; such as disturbed sleep pattern, lethargy, exhaustion and anxiety. The patient in denial may be an expert in colluding with those around him, including the physician to support the conviction that they need a holiday, a rest from work or a change of job. If depression is suggested to be the possible cause of symptoms, it is rigorously dismissed. Powerful defense mechanisms will be in place to discourage or cut dead even the suggestion of depressive illness. For some, even the barest suggestion of depressive illness may send the visiting patient scurrying off to try out an assortment of deflective pursuits; anything from doing a college course, going to the gym, or seeking out the help of alternative health practitioners, all of whom may serve to alleviate the depression temporarily at the best. Physical exercise is a known method of intervention for depression, as it stimulates cortical functioning in the brain. Cognitive Behavior Therapy (CBT) explicitly targets this area of the brain. For example, embarking on a college course which stimulates cortical activity can be known to soothe anxious thoughts.

Even though antidepressants in the 1980s, in the form of Prozac and Seroxat, were less riddled with unpleasant side effects, people were still reluctant to admit they were taking antidepressants, even though they might have painlessly crossed the threshold from being medication-free to taking medication with relative ease.

The insights of sociologist David Karp are important here when describing the protracted and often painful process that leads to taking medication. He refers to this as an 'evolution in illness consciousness' which is manifested through four successive stages. These are:

Resistance
Trial Commitment
Conversion
Disenchantment

Resistance manifests in the form of what I have been writing about where denial, ambivalence and anger towards one's own powerlessness keep one away from medication. Various other reasons would be a concern about the long-term implications of taking medication based on information from colleagues, friends and family. Additionally, the media has a tendency to highlight the negatives and horror stories linked with prescriptive medication, rather than the lives it has saved and brought back from the brink. Making that step from being a relatively healthy, albeit, haunted individual, to realizing that one has an illness, calls for a redefinition of the self as mentally unstable, if not psychologically challenged.

Trial commitment often asserts itself at a later stage where, through unacceptable behavior in the form of self-harm (more common in women) and violence in men, sends them along to a recommended psychiatrist. Often, medication only becomes allowed in when, through no fault of their own, the depressed person finds themselves in a psychiatric hospital after ending up in Casualty with an overdose. Alternatively, when finding oneself recuperating from a hangover and a painful encounter with some unforgiving wall, or locked up in a police cell again; one is persuaded to see a psychiatrist. It is at this point of sobering confinement that the depressed person may receive their first real diagnosis. On an initial first meeting with a psychiatrist the depressive may receive their first real diagnosis which can be both a relief and a shock. A regime of treatment in the form of medication and attending a group session with other sufferers, may make it possible to redefine oneself in a supportive environment.

After the treatment package has had time to work and the patient has received all the support they need to help them through a wobbly period, they may be discharged from hospital with their medication and several follow-up visits to the psychiatrist or a weekly visit from a Community Psychiatric Nurse (CPN). With the help of their physician or psychiatrist the patient gradually tapers off medication and returns to work, if they have any. With the loss of medical and psychiatric support and the stress of getting back to work various stress triggers will come into play; creating stress on top of stress in the form of panic attacks and growing anxiety. This transitional period of getting back to normal life can be negotiated successfully, but after a failed attempt and lacking a proper support network, the convalescent will go back onto medication and perhaps be on it indefinitely. Depression caused by bereavement or an emotional setback of some kind or, in the face of important exams, usually responds well to a short period of medication. Here, their efficacy in addressing a short-term problem and their subsequent withdrawal is irrefutable. Alternatively, a depressed person may be on medication for some months, even a couple of years, and hit a period of feeling 'better than well' – which is quite common in the summer months. Independently, they reach a decision to give up their medication as this case history of a young girl in her early 20s illustrates:

I'd been on antidepressants for a couple of years and had been feeling very good. I had a new boyfriend and was doing well in my job and I just thought giving up the tablets was the right thing to do. I skipped doses then dropped them all together and still felt fine. But after a few weeks things began to get me down and irritate me and I thought it was work. Then my boyfriend dumped me – and suddenly I was rock bottom.

The next thing I knew I woke up in Casualty and they were pumping my stomach because I had taken an overdose. I only vaguely remember taking those pills. Obviously I had to agree to see the Shrink and before I knew it I was sectioned and spent three weeks in a psychiatric hospital...

I'm back on medication now and feel okay again... I have to tell myself that it is dangerous to go off medication too suddenly, if at all...

This case history is not dissimilar to many others. In my hospital working environment there are usually at least half a dozen patients on any medical ward who suffer from underlying depression. It isn't unusual to have one patient who has taken an overdose on a ward at any given time awaiting psychiatric review. I would say that a large amount of the patients have stopped medication prior to taking the overdose. I have to point out here, that it is not coming off medication that can trigger a suicidal state, but the sudden cessation of medication altogether can leave the patient vulnerable to mood swings and weaken one's ability to tackle challenging life situations. Life is stressful enough as it is, but for people especially vulnerable to any additional stress, withdrawing from medication too quickly can be the trigger that sends one over the edge.

There are three main types of antidepressants available today; the *Tricyclics*, *MAOIs* and the newer 'cleaner' ones, the SSRIs. They are all 70% effective if taken properly, have various side effects that may be helpful to some people, and less helpful to others and all are targeted to act on several neurotransmitters that have a direct effect on mood and bodily functions.

Most people are concerned about how addictive drugs are; becoming stuck on them forever, or their side effects. And here I want to include my own experience of medication alongside valuable research and direct contact with other people.

Antidepressants, in themselves, are not addictive in the same way as the benzodiazepines such as Valium and Librium can be. But, because they can make you feel well, you may feel that you don't need them anymore. And this may be so, but often a sudden break with medication can bring about a relapse. Giving up medication should be done slowly and incrementally. I have met an alarming amount of patients who have stopped their medication too quickly and ended up in hospital as a result of a suicide attempt or other acts of self-harm. A sudden relapse can be more distressing than the actual symptoms of depression. It should be remembered that depression is a serious, debilitating condition as potentially life-threatening as diabetes, cardiac problems, and cancer. Sometimes, just feeling well can be a sign that the medication is working! The guilt about taking medication may need to be addressed rather than the efficacy of any certain drug. Furthermore, the decision to take medication can bring up all sorts of issues around pride, autonomy, control and ambivalence towards being dependent on a chemical substance.

Tolerance can be mistaken for addiction in that, with time, the body becomes acclimatized to a particular medication, so more is needed. Increasing the dose may be effective and legitimate for a while, until a decision is made between you and your physician whether you want to continue increasing the dose or try something else. Since everyone is different, there is no guarantee that a drug will cease to be effective with time. Some people can take a medication for a number of years without having to increase their medication or change it. One of the main precursors to medication failing or not being as effective as it could be, are increasing stress levels in the person's life. Even when you are well and perhaps, *especially* so, because your defenses are down, you are vulnerable to stress.

It is not possible to discuss medication without including your physician because their experience, insight, understanding or lack of it will influence your choice. Like anything, there are doctors that are sympathetic and have more than a perfunctory interest in depression, and there are others who are unsympathetic and antagonistic towards mental illness. To be fair, physicians are not psychiatrists, but they are expected to be because of the one-in-four depressed people who enter their surgery. A doctor who is honest about his own shortcomings in this area can be infinitely more helpful by referring his depressed patients to a psychiatrist rather than imposing mindsets on those who have come to him for help. The problem is that depression can be either precipitated by psychological problems or biological ones or a combination of both. I have to say that for someone who has moved about a lot, abroad and in this country, there are excellent physicians about who have an understanding of the magnitude of depressive illness. These, I have found, have either admitted to depressive illness themselves or have had relations, colleagues or close friends who suffer from it. The physician I have now, although not suffering from depression himself, firmly believes that many people suffer from a serotonin deficiency. Although he does not suffer from depression himself, he is aware of its gravity through his fellow colleagues, friends and even family members. By the same token, there are sympathetic psychiatrists and less sympathetic psychiatrists.

The inclusion of the 'healing field' here is of paramount importance when visiting a representative of the medical profession. We may need to remind ourselves that the person sitting behind the desk is more than a label, but a human being and a soul whom we have invited to travel with us on our journey. I have always found that including the situation in the healing field creates the right ambience for the meeting with 'experts' who can otherwise seem daunting. Often, it is not what is or isn't said in the consulting room but in the unspoken silence. Remember, if we go in to see the doctor or expert with mindsets based on preconceived ideas or history the 'other' will respond to these mindsets in their own way. The diagnosis of a condition although informed by knowledge and skill is also dependent on intuition coming to the fore as well. Mindsets and resentments can seriously impede the flow of intuition. Like anything, going for a consultation to a representative of their field, whether it is medical, psychiatric or business is part of a process. We can enable the process to come into being by being conscious of the 'space' we are creating. Just because we may have had a negative experience in the past with a doctor or psychiatrist doesn't mean this is going to be the same within the next encounter.

I want to briefly cover the three types of medication used in treating depression along with their benefits and common side effects.

SSRIs (Selective Serotonin Reuptake Inhibitors)
Prozac has been the star and forerunner of the SSRIs which came onto the market in the 1980s. Basically, they inhibit the neuro-transmitter, serotonin, from being taken up by the body too quickly, by keeping the serotonin in the synaptic cleft for a longer period. In this way receptors at the end of the neurons have more opportunity to absorb and pass on the chemical. In depressed people there is usually a faulty serotonergic system that prevents serotonin from being passed between the nerve cells efficiently.

Although serotonin has been targeted by the earlier tricyclic antidepressants, the SSRIs because of their fine tuning have less likelihood of toxic side effects. For this reason, they are often the preferred medication when prescribing for potentially suicidal patients. Additionally, besides alleviating depression, they are found helpful for young people with various psychological conditions like self-harming, anorexia nervosa and Obsessive Compulsive Disorder (OCD), anxiety and personality disorders.

SSRIs include Prozac (fluoextine),Seroxat (paroxetine), Lustral (sertraline) and Cipramil (citalpram). Prozac's popularity has been largely due to the fact that its side effects are few and it seems to be an all-rounder. It is extremely effective in mobilizing energy and releasing one's 'get-up and go'. I took Prozac for two years and apart from an initial adaptation period of a few weeks I have found it by far the best medication for me. It pulled me from the brink of suicide and despair. I felt more myself than I had in some years. I can honestly say that without Prozac's efficacy, I would not be alive today. Although I have to add, because of my level of despair, it took six weeks to become fully effective! The speed at which medication takes to become fully effective depends on each patient and the particular medication.

There are far fewer side effects with SSRIs than with other types of antidepressants, once the adaptation period has been negotiated. The initial and more common sensations are nausea, loss of appetite, dizziness and feeling spaced out. Also, like most antidepressants, there may be disturbances in libido.

There has been a lot of negative publicity towards the SSRIs — the main reason being that they can evoke suicidal feelings, especially in the early stages. I feel I want to add here that in deep depression often it is impossible to find the will to mobilize and act out any disturbing feelings. The critical stage, as all psychiatrists and most physicians know is at that point where the depressed person is beginning to get better and feelings are flooding back. And this is why it is important for a healthcare professional to closely monitor their patient's progress.

Incidentally, the hidden benefits of SSRIs, particularly Prozac, is their ability to promote neurogenesis; the growth of new brain cells. This has got to be a good thing as deep and prolonged depression has been medically proven to cause brain tissue to atrophy. Additionally, similar to the tricyclics, they have a positive effect on alleviating irritable bowel syndrome.

Tricyclics
These have been around a lot longer than the SSRIs and were developed in the 1950s. Their name is derived from their molecular constitution in which the atom was made up of three rings. The tricyclics work by inhibiting the re-uptake of the neurotransmitters norepinephrine, dopamine or serotonin by nerve cells.

The first one to emerge by chance was Iproniazid which was a drug used initially in the treatment of tuberculosis. While improving appetite and generally aiding the constitution it was noticed that people who took it became 'inappropriately happy'. Iproniazid became used as one of the first effective anti-depressants marketed in 1958. It was regarded as a psychic energizer.

The calming sedative effects are experienced immediately, and they are highly effective where depression is anxiety based. Despite the recent advent of SSRIs the tricyclics are still popular with many older people. The main ones are Dothiepin,

Clomapramil and Amytriptiline. Dothiepin was my first introduction to an effective antidepressant and I found it very helpful
for some months in both calming me and enabling me to sleep
when my stress levels were very high.

Initial side effects are blurred vision, dry mouth, drowsiness
and difficulty urinating. These symptoms may persist as dosage
is increased.

The hidden benefits of the tricyclics are in their various pain-
relieving qualities especially in neuromuscular pain and in alleviating irritable bowel syndrome.

Monoamine Oxidase Inhibitors (MAOIs): is an enzyme found
in the human body which, in the brain, breaks down neurotransmitters such as serotonin and norepinephrine. Putting the brakes
on this enzyme's action raises the level of neurotransmitters
which, in turn, elevate the mood. Although they are highly
effective, because of their toxic interaction with certain foods,
they are not always first choice of antidepressant. Yet, they are
sometimes used as a last resort for those resistant to the tricyclics
and SSRIs. The foods they interact with are ones containing the
amino acid, tyramine, which can contribute to high blood
pressure. Since tyramine is found in red wine, particularly
Chianti, liver, fava beans, marmite and other yeast-based
spreads, it poses a sustained vigilance on what one eats which
might not always be possible in the face of debilitating illness.
These older drugs include Phenalzine and Parnate. With the
advent of newer MAOIs there are fewer side effects. More
recently a patch can be worn so absorption doesn't interfere with
digestion.

MAOIs are particularly effective for depression when there
are symptoms of overeating, sleeplessness and anxiety. One of
their hidden benefits is their ability in curbing the desire to
smoke.

As in all antidepressant medication it is important that they
are not mixed and, if they are, that this is done on the advice of a

physician or psychiatrist who is aware of the various contra-indications.

Lithium

This is the lightest of the solid elements and, because of this, is believed to have possessed 'modest magical qualities.'

Although lithium carbonate has been around since the 1940s and, as in, so many successful chemicals was discovered largely by chance. It is used, very effectively, today in the treatment of bipolar disorder. It is a natural salt of glutamic acid, the main excitatory neurotransmitter for all nerve impulses in the mammalian brain. Its role here has been to stabilize the mood swings from suicidal depression to mania. American Psychiatrist, Kay Redfield Jamison, praises its efficacy both in her own life in treating her bipolar disorder but also its use as an anti-suicide medication. She believes its efficacy is due to the "capacity to enhance serotonin turnover in the brain" as well as aiding the efficacy of other neurotransmitters. As an end result of this, there is a decrease in aggression, agitation, depression and mania.

I talked with a friend recently who suffered from bipolar disorder and had been on lithium for several years. He likened it to a seatbelt he needed to wear when he was traveling through life. He described it as keeping him just short of flying too high or, falling like the mythical Icarus, back into the sea. He explained how it just kept his chin above the floor when he plunged into a downward spiral.

Although lithium works very well, it does need to be monitored regularly through routine blood tests as too little of it can be ineffective and too higher a dose can be toxic. By the same token, it does not necessarily suit everyone, although there are many claims that it can be a miracle drug. A study in the late 1990s in Sweden revealed that, statistically, there was as much as a 77% reduction in suicide when taking lithium. This is quite remarkable.

Side Effects

Although it is important we don't become overwhelmed by the possible side effects of a medication, it is common sense accepting that there will be some initial side effects while the medication is entering into the bodily system. That is why a relatively low and ineffective dose is introduced initially. Side effects can be equated with a new pair of glasses or contact lenses which we need to familiarize ourselves with, or the supportive arches in a pair of shoes. Anything new often exacerbates the underlying condition initially rather than make it better.

To look at side effects more realistically we should not isolate this from the side effects or collateral we can suffer when we do anything different. Medication is by no means isolated in this. If we go to the gym after a long period of inactivity or take up jogging, we will experience aching and sore muscles until our body acclimatizes to the new form of exercise. Acclimatization to a new altitude is often worse in the first few weeks. If we take up studying after a long period away, we will experience tiredness and the sense of being overwhelmed by the sheer volume of information until our bodily system adapts. Similarly, if we take up full-time work again after a long break we are bound to feel stressed and exhausted for the first few weeks until we become familiar with the working environment. Because we have an innate dislike for these unpleasant side effects we may become discouraged after the first few weeks and convince ourselves that the bad effects outweigh the good and give up. In order to continue an activity that appears to be taking more out of us then we are getting back, it is important to keep aligned to *purpose, meaning* and *values*. Just one of these life-saving qualities will enable us to find the will to carry it through. If our purpose, in this context, is to feel less depressed, we have to put up with the initial side effects such as increased anxiety or feeling sedated. Most of the time, it will pass, and this is why any physician will advise we call back in ten days after we have commenced the medication in order to monitor our progress. The first two weeks are the critical phase where we may actually feel worse before we feel better. This is also true of many complementary therapies such as homeopathy or reflexology when we may actually feel worse to begin with, or other deep seated problems may resurface. These are side effects too. Initial ones that pass as time goes by.

Basically, all antidepressants take time to have a tangible positive effect. This can be anything from 10 days to 6 weeks. If one is in a critical state of depression and cannot tolerate waiting for such a long period because of high levels of anxiety making sleeping and eating impossible, the psychiatrist might prescribe a short period of tranquillizers until the anti-depressants have kicked in. Providing the patient isn't suicidal, this can be a very reliable way to make things run more smoothly. I have experienced this passage into antidepressants myself and found it very effective and did not feel addicted in any way after the tranquillizers had run their course. This saved me a lot of unbearable anxiety.

Why Medication Doesn't Always Work

Any psychiatrist will say that one of the reasons why medication doesn't always work is because only 3 out of 5 people follow the instructions. The advice here is to *give them a chance to work!*

Reasons for this are because people think they can self-medicate; for example they might begin to feel worse and after a few days discontinue the tablets. Others may feel ashamed of taking medication and cut down indiscriminately to make themselves feel better about taking them. I have known people resort to just taking one antidepressant *now* and *then!* Sadly, antidepressants are not like narcotics or tranquilizers with an immediate effect. Still others will, after feeling better, give up their medication thinking they are cured. Another simple reason why medication may not work is because the dose is not high enough for the person, or in some cases is too high.

Sometimes doctors that have no real empathy or understanding of the condition will get someone to cut down before they are ready, putting them on a maintenance dose. In this sense, not all doctors know what they are doing. I have found the wiser ones will admit this and enter into dialogue with the patient and their relatives so that it can be a shared responsibility.

And here I do want to stress the importance of having a mentor or friend with you when visiting your physician. In this way, the depressive whose mental, emotional and psychological factors are greatly reduced has the support of a mentor. This is basically someone who knows and understands the patient and can fill in important details of the condition which may be easily overlooked in the midst of a stressful situation where time is in short supply.

The other reason why medication doesn't always work is because the medication may not suit the person or can interact adversely with other medication. Like anything, getting the right medication and dosage is a process of trial-and-error which requires patience and persistence.

What to do when Medication does Work

Stay on the medication!

Although this may be obvious, it is amazing how many people decide it's time to jack in a course of treatment which may be actually working! This is like sailing into calmer waters after a terrifying storm and then, after no time at all to reassess the situation, or draw up preventative measures, go heading straight out into the storm again!

And it is worth remembering here that rather than medication being a last resort or the end of the road, it may actually mark the beginning of accepting better health and a stability which enables long-term plans to be made. Making long-term plans may not have been possible before. Certainly, this has been true for me.

Since, in the face of depression, happiness and joy can be so elusive, I want to include them here as they are woven very closely to both bipolar disorder and depression itself. Additionally, as human beings, we are primed to seek happiness and joy. But what is the distinction between the two?

Chapter 8

The Anatomy of Joy and Happiness

When we are no longer able to change a situation, we are challenged to change ourselves.
Viktor Frankl, prisoner and Camp Psychiatrist in Belson

The symbol for the I-Ching with its two interlocking half circles, one black and the other white could represent the interface of joy and happiness. In a sense, joy is a higher octave of happiness.

Joy, unlike happiness, is something the world can neither give nor take away.

Like a living barometer, our mood bobs up and down with fluctuations of thought, interaction with others, or simply – the weather. Happiness, like sadness, tends to be transitory according to our moods or how we meet everyday experience. We can be reading a book and if we get involved with the central character, our moods fluctuate with the moods of the characters as we identify with them. Sometimes there are mixed feelings as in a combination of happiness and sadness. For example, I experience a joy when I witness the arrival of house martins, arctic terns and eider ducks on the Cumbrian peninsular where I live. Each time they arrive, I am thrilled they have made it, again, across sea and land. But then I experience a sadness when they start to gather on the telephone lines in musical notes, chattering excitedly as they prepare to leave. I have mixed feelings when I witness their tenacity of purpose. Yet, I know that they will take the last vestiges of summer with them on their long flight home and this fills me with mixed feelings, of happiness and sadness.

Although happiness and joy are often used interchangeably, they are as different to each other as black and white. Happiness originates from the root word 'hap' which means chance or fate.

Joy is a higher octave of happiness because it is more potent, more consuming, more sought after because it is elusive. The Thesaurus interprets joy as 'bliss', 'blessedness and beatitude'.

Perhaps, this is why happiness is more accessible than joy because we can engage in activities which make us happy, such as going to a restaurant for dinner, watching a film or taking a holiday. But happiness is rarely constant. As soon as we think we have it, it slips away like seed fluff, eluding us completely. We glimpse this in the transparency of children who are longing for the latest computer game or film. The longing is actually in the *waiting*, the anticipation. When they have received the object of their desire, their initial enthusiasm ebbs away after a short time as they go on to seek some other new novelty.

It is not surprising that one of the most challenging tasks in life is maintaining an inner sense of equilibrium. When we are young, we are easily swayed from one extreme emotion to another as we are pulled by the kaleidoscope of temptations which demand our attention. Feelings are volatile and thoughts so mercurial that sometimes it seems too much to bear. Alcohol can seem the only escape from all the things demanding our attention, but relief is short and addictive. Harder still, is the call to actualize our potential – become who we are born to be. It can be easier to close down what is struggling to be born in us in order to fit in. Sometimes it seems that there is no choice but to follow the crowd. Yet, in this betrayal of our value in the world, we invite the Black Dog to take up residence in our life.

Yet, the truth is, whatever situation we are in, we *always* have choice. We may not feel this is so, but until we do, we cannot grow in psychological or emotional maturity. By our outlook we define whether our emotional wings are spread out ready to fly or are cauterized. But, in order to grow into the soul of the world, it may be necessary to undergo a level of suffering. I am reminded here of the words of psychiatrist and author, Viktor Frankl: 'What is to give light, must endure burning'.

Frankl, as a Jew, was imprisoned for three years in a Nazi prisoner-of-war camp where he endured hard labor and then was moved to Bergen/Belson and sentenced to another seven months' hard labor. Yet, amidst this, he had a positive effect on the prisoners. His words imparted hope to all the other inmates—where there had been none before. Realizing his value, his jailors appointed him to Camp Psychiatrist. Frankl understood the value of meaning, perhaps more than anyone. He believed that if people failed to experience a sense of meaning in their everyday life and, in this sense, within the confines of the prison camp, they were likely to give up and perish without hope. Above all, he believed that if a person could live in the present, rather than zoning out to another preferred time and place, they would not lose the will to carry on. Living in the past, as so many prisoners did, rendered them unable to see value and opportunity in the present. It was through utilizing the opportunity in the moment, that meaning could be found. He utilized this outlook as a springboard to develop his greatest work ever and which he called Existential Psychology. After his release, he taught this in Vienna.

Although our personal circumstances are unlikely to be as dire as this, awareness of how the mind works can serve us well in our daily life. Instead of unconscious, reactive choices we can make informed, conscious choices. After all, the choices we make, define who we are.

Similarly, in the depths of my own depression, like many people, I was able to access and express creatively what gave my life meaning, in the form of my writing. It isn't always understood that art and invention are not necessarily the product of happiness and satisfaction but, rather through loss, hardship and anguish. It kept me alive, kept me going – a little bit each day like those underground tunnels prisoners-of-war painstakingly chiseled out to escape their incarceration. It wasn't that my writing in itself gave me hope. It didn't. Rather, it sustained those three vital qualities which connect us to our vision in life: *value*, *meaning* and *purpose*. These qualities, rather like the mythological Ariadne's thread, which would keep Theseus on course to finding his way back out of the labyrinth after slaying the Minotaur.

My wish that burned like a light throughout my inner incarceration was that, one day, my experience of depression would be of value to others throughout their silent and hidden dis-ease of being. No one can really understand depression unless they have had experienced it personally or through a family member or close friend.

The late archetypal psychologist, James Hillman, often referred to the value of soul-making which is a term used by John Keats for our human condition in the world:

Building the psychic vessel of containment, which is another way of speaking of soul making, seems to require bleeding and leaking as its precondition. Why else go through that work unless we are driven by the despair of our unstoppered condition?

And—so I have come full circle! In a chapter titled 'Happiness and joy' sadness and suffering have slipped into the text. Yet, like that I-Ching symbol of Yin and Yang and black and white, they are inseparable as the shadow is from the sun, or the brilliance of the stars from the night sky. It is interesting how little I have written about joy, as if saving it for last, rather than consuming it first.

This provides a clue to which level we are addressing in our understanding of joy. Unlike happiness, joy lacks a tangible image to connect to such as a new car, a new boyfriend or a new house. We cannot order joy, snatch at it, pin it down or buy it. Joy is never up for sale, although it may be evoked by a scene or person. Rather, it is an invisible quality which graces us, pays homage to us, unbidden. It may arrive in the form of a sunset or wild geese flying across the dawn sky. It is as if some magical casement and like the boy in the *Secret Garden* we find a whole new world. We are in awe.

Juxtaposed between this sense of fantasy and acute reality we feel vibrantly alive and whole. Because joy is brief but incredibly intense, it becomes imprinted on our memory template. Unlike the barometer of happiness which goes up and down with our moods, joy is something that rises up within us spontaneously, as if it was always there, yet something sparked it into awareness.

It is like the dragonfly larva which lies at the bottom of a muddy pool for months, years even, then one day emerges to realize its potential in the form of this exquisite creature of winged beauty. It *is* a miracle!

Joy too, is a miracle because, unlike happiness, we cannot *make* it happen. It is innate in us, emerging every now and then into our consciousness to make us feel connected to our potential, the world and all those people around us. Herein lies a deeper lesson in not judging anything by its appearance. Because, when we do, we close down to the miracle it can become. It is the same with depression, when we experience the pull of gravity and long to break free from this very real sense of imprisonment, we may fail to harness its potential. Depression offers a steep learning curve to all those that are affected by it. Like the transformation of the dragonfly from an ugly grub, understanding how to siphon the value of it from the wreckage it leaves behind is of paramount importance. Certainly, the media which has become a God in itself, very rarely sheds light on its value. Depression, like all dis-ease of the body, mind and soul, holds the rich potential for transformation into meaning, purpose and value... And, in this context—joy!

Joy is infectious. It affects everyone, reminding me of the white choir of snowdrops which suddenly reveal themselves through the hedgerows in the early spring. Although most of us have had a joyful experience or several within our lifetime, it rarely gets talked about. It is too precious. Instead, it is stored deep within us, very rarely emerging into the consciousness of everyday life. Yet, it is sought after as fervently as the mystics of old sought after the magical elixir which transmutes base metals into gold. Although joy is spontaneous, unlike happiness, we cannot make it happen, because it is there already. Eastern teachings inform us that all the material distractions of the world mask the real truth which is drinking from an infinite well of internal joy. Yet, paradoxically, we have an inbuilt longing for bliss, so we plunder the world, substituting inner joy for outer happiness.

I am reminded here of a time in my early 30s when I was traveling from Euston station to Manchester Piccadilly and there were few seats on the train which were not reserved or taken. But my gaze kept being drawn towards one table seat next to an Asian family dressed in their brightly colored saris. The young mother and baby beamed at me as I took the spare seat. We began to talk. They were just returning from visiting their family members in Delhi to their home in Manchester. The baby girl sitting on her mother's lap was about a year old with caramel-colored eyes and a ready smile.

"What is her name?" I asked.

"Joy," the mother responded, "Would you like to hold her?"

"Yes, I'd love to…"

Joy beamed at me as I took her and sat her on my lap. "Joy?" I repeated. 'What a lovely name!'

The pleasure I experienced holding this baby was so spontaneous and beautiful that I will never forget it… especially as I had recently emerged from six months of debilitating depression.

Exercise for Tapping into your Joy

I want to say here that joy does not have to be attached to anything concrete or physical. For example, my first conscious moment of joy took place when I was nine years old. It was early one Sunday morning with the sun enticing me through my bedroom window. Suddenly, I decided to climb out of the bedroom window of the bungalow where I lived, not wanting to wake anyone else.

My walk took me through several public gardens where it would lead me onto the promenade overlooking the sea. The appeal was in the fact that no one was about and I felt it was 'my time'. Dew covered the grasses in the gardens, each blade embroidered in a scintillating tapestry of flame-colored jewels. Within this amphitheater of magic, I walked through the gardens, experiencing the rich birdsong sounding about me. At that time of day and in the 1960s there was very little noise pollution about.

You will probably find that your memories will return to you in images because they are, as Freud intimated, the language of the unconscious. Questions always open up consciousness so that memories are more accessible.

Allow yourself to return to your early memories of childhood
Can you remember when you experienced your first memory of joy?
Where were you at the time?
What were you doing at the time?
It doesn't matter whether you were passive or active. Joy is joy and, unlike happiness, isn't necessarily evoked by physical action.
Were you on your own? If not, where were you and who were you with?
Can you remember what age you were when you first experienced joy?
What did the joy look like? Can you find an image for it or a scent or color?
What age were you?
Was this joy elicited by something you were given?
Or was it something you found for yourself?
If you like, make more notes or sketch an image of it.

Questions speak directly to the unconscious.

They evoke traces of the past like the contrails left behind by aircraft. It is important that questions are asked in order to bypass the concrete brain and invite what is held in the unconscious to become conscious. And the question I want to leave you with is this:

How did your initial experiences of joy impact on you later in your life?

Above all, don't worry if your mind is a blank and it seems impossible to access the information from your past memories. The unconscious, once activated by questions, will work overtime and visit you in your dreams and in sudden insights throughout the day. An image may come, but instead of pushing it away, allow it to speak to you. It is worth keeping pen and paper by your bed so that you can capture it in words. It doesn't matter how clear images from the unconscious can appear to be, if not committed to paper, they will slip away like dew in the morning sun. The act of writing and drawing creates a connection in the brain so that a neural pathway is laid down. Piaget, the child psychologist, knew the wisdom of connecting the brain with the body. He understood that the act of manipulating objects with the hands feeds and creates neural pathways in the brain which strengthen and grow as the child masters and acts on his environment. Like many people who are concerned about education solely through computers, I wonder how much our electronic- and data-defined world will impact on the young child's development.

Chapter 9

Crisis and Leadership

Some of our best and most successful world leaders have been shadowed by mental illness and, in the context of this book, major depression. To further illustrate this, I am wanting to look at the lives of two well-known political leaders; the first being our iconic Winston Churchill, the second, the former US president, Abraham Lincoln, the 16th president of the United States.

Although Churchill referred frequently to his well-known 'Black Dog' in connection with depression, the usage of this metaphor actually preceded Churchill by several hundred years. Primarily used in the 1700s, it actually came into usage with Dr Samuel Johnson, an English Lexicographer, who used this expression to describe his own melancholia. He believed that depression never really leaves his master, because it 'dogs' him. It is both diligent and faithful in its behavior. Before that, in the fifth century BC, Hippocrates, the father of modern medicine, defined depression as 'melancholia', known also as 'Black Bile'. Hippocrates asserted that the seat of all thought and emotional illness resided in the brain. In a sense, he made depression respectable and, in his own words 'a long labor of the soul can produce melancholy.'

Perhaps this is why depression has always been associated with highly creative people, particularly poets, musicians, artists, writers and inventors such as Isaac Newton who also suffered from depression.

Returning to Churchill, he was described as belligerent, outspoken and brilliant. It seemed that he needed very little sleep, which is one of the defining symptoms of manic depressive illness. And yet – he was successful in his task, in fact, outstanding.

I also believe he worked with his intuition because he sensed the very real danger the Germans would place the British in long before his fellow politicians. He believed war was imminent. Yet, his call to invest in military spending was turned down by his own cousin, Lord Londonderry. He adamantly resisted all Churchill's efforts to invest in expanding British air forces.

Psychiatrist, Nassir Ghaemi, author of *A Fine Madness*, explores the link between fine leadership and mental illness. Furthermore, he asserts that in relatively stable times, political leaders do well in 'sailing the ship of State' on course. Critical and unstable times, such as being at war, calls for another type of leadership altogether—one that takes risks and doesn't tread the well-known way for the sake of maintaining the status quo. Certainly, Churchill fitted this bill.

Ghaemi cites qualities which moderate to severely depressed people possess in the form of resilience, empathy, creativity and realism. Many innovators and leaders can become star-struck by their own ideas and sense of importance and lose sight of the ground beneath their feet. In stark contrast, depressed leaders come to the fore in turmoil and danger. Because so much of their life has been challenging, they possess the sort of emotional and mental resilience necessary for maintaining their vision and bringing it into form. Also, they are not easily dissuaded by obstacles and setbacks and, if anything, are motivated by adversity.

Abraham Lincoln, perhaps known best for abolishing the slave trade, became president of the United States in 1860. He emerged from a poor background and was raised in a log cabin in Kentucky with very little schooling so that he was self-educated. He was also used to adversity from a very early age, particularly from his father who was resentful and ambivalent towards him and thought nothing of regularly beating him.

Lincoln also suffered from suicidal depression from a very early age. Fortunately he had a clutch of very good friends who took turns at keeping him on 'suicide watch' on several occasions. Both Lincoln and Churchill are well-known historical figures who, despite their unenviable contract with depression, utilized their 'black dog' as a foundation to become highly original and powerful leaders. There are many other leaders who similarly, suffer from unremitting depression who, although not necessarily on a political level, become creative and well-respected people. Depression itself is not a lost cause. Unlike many other forms of physical and mental suffering, it can be used as a foundation to create a powerful caste for a work of value. For example and in the context of this work, many pioneers in the medical profession suffer from depression themselves. To support this, I am thinking here of psychiatrists and psychologists whose work I have become familiar with through my research. Kay Redfield Jamison, author of the well-researched book *Touched with fire*, an iconic work about well-known creative people, suffered from bipolar depression herself. Also, Martha Manning, a psychologist, who chronicles twenty months of her life in the book, *Undercurrents*. Andrew Solomon, journalist and author has written a highly informative tome on the nature and history of depression in *The Noonday Demon* together with his own experiences. Here he writes about his own descent into depression in his 40s. Journalist, Mark Rice-Oxley, author of *Underneath the Lemon Tree*, writes cogently about his disintegration into darkness at the age of 40. These examples define a cross-section of highly intelligent people who, despite their knowledge, career success and strong social network, became suddenly enveloped by a depression which was relentless and unforgiving.

As historical narratives reveal, no one is immune to depression. It undermines all sectors of society, all ages irrespective of class, money or education. It can be hereditary, but not necessarily so. One of the qualities of conscious suffering in any shape or form is empathy. This is frequently often underpinned by a willingness to help others who suffer from the same condition. An example of this is Abraham Lincoln's empathy for the imprisoned slaves so endemic of the time in which he lived. Perhaps their imprisonment mirrored his own sense of being incarcerated within the unforgiving prison of his own illness.

Empathy and compassion are valued qualities in the healthcare profession. Without them there is no real understanding or patience for those clients/patients within their care. Following this line of thought, many physicians who have either suffered from depression themselves or been affected by a family member or close friend with it, are less likely to pass it off as a symptom of weakness. Similarly, a person who has experienced depression and refused to look into the reasons why, perhaps escaping through alcohol or drugs, is in danger of projecting their fear onto others who talk about it openly, and deride their experiences. Yet, to be fair, underpinning this unforgiving outlook, we only have to explore our cultural and historical mindsets to understand why. Early methods of intervention in sanatoriums ranged from bloodletting, holding subjects underwater until they almost drowned, spinning stools to induce dizziness in an effort to eject 'spirits' and forced-feeding were frequently carried out in sanatoriums for depressed people. Is it any surprise that this endemic ostracism of mental illness has built up a formidable legacy of shame and self-loathing over the years?

Since a physician is the first person you approach if you feel desperate enough to seek help, one would expect or hope the doctor approached would have some insight into such a common illness.

After a basic appraisal of your state of health and family history, they might set up a package of counseling together with the intervention of medication to initiate the healing process. I have been fortunate in later years to have a physician who treated me with the respect and dignity that you would expect. But this has not always been the case.

Here is my experience of two physicians I approached with depression:

Dr Maws, a youngish doctor, crossed his legs uncomfortably and avoided eye contact when I described my symptoms. I had finally plucked up the courage to visit a doctor in the vicinity where I had just moved to. After glancing at me briefly, he asked me what I did. I explained as best as I could that I was a Clinical Support Worker in a busy hospital environment.

"No wonder, you're depressed—working with the sick and dying," he remarked coldly. "Can't you do something else?"

I was speechless as I stared back at him in dismay. Wasn't he working with the sick and dying himself? Was this the sort of biased advice he was giving to all his depressed patients? When I told him, trying desperately to hold back the tears and escape the chasm that had opened up inside me, he turned on me.

"Well!" he said. "You've got yourself into a right state! Haven't you?"

On the heels of that, he told me to come off my antidepressants 'cold turkey' instead of tapering the dose off incrementally or even starting me on something different.

Anyone familiar with antidepressants will know that it can be dangerous to stop them abruptly without slowly introducing a new drug. The side effects of coming off *Effexor* cold turkey were relentless and protracted. Although, in the 1990s, there was some awareness of this in the medical profession along with a validation of the 'head zapping' withdrawal effects, this knowledge obviously didn't extend to Doctor Maws.

Today, withdrawal symptoms are validated as a genuine response to a sudden cessation in medication, frequently referred to as 'discontinuation syndrome'. I had what is called 'head zaps' which feel like electrical shocks being administered to the brain. Additionally, I had vertigo and dizziness which would last for hours. I had to give up work for some weeks, losing pay, because I was unable to function, let alone go to work. But, on the advice of a close friend, I cut down on my medication, incrementally, week by week which suited me better. The drug companies didn't want to admit to physical withdrawal symptoms at the time. That came later, after a number of suicides pressured the drug companies to release information based on their grueling experiences; these were added to the list of side effects amongst a proposed percentage of 'users'. At the time, I was feeling suicidal and if it wasn't for the support of a close friend, I am pretty sure I would have ended it. Of course, and to be fair, not everyone has withdrawal symptoms, but *large* amounts *do*. This is supported by a number of incidents where people coming off certain antidepressants too quickly became suicidal and were admitted to hospital as emergencies.

Fortunately, I had a positive experience with another doctor in the practice who was older, wiser and empathic rather than defensive. Dr Ruby validated my experience and indirectly referred to other patients who had suffered similar side effects. Immediately, I felt at ease. He asked me if I was suicidal and said if I was, he would have to admit me to a psychiatric hospital in Whitehaven. I didn't perceive this frank comment as a threat but rather a sensible solution to what could be a dramatic outcome. First and foremost, Dr Ruby saw me as a person presenting mental, emotional and physical symptoms of depression. He saw me as a human being in distress and realized I needed immediate medical intervention.

Although depression is widespread, there is an irrational fear of it and this attitude underpins the cultural mindset that depression is to be feared and exiled from the population. What you are afraid of, you shut the door on. Depression is not contagious. However, what it does magnify is our powerlessness in being able to fix it or snap out of it. I think, underpinning this, is the knowledge that depression runs like unwelcome tributaries through every class and cross-section of society, young and old, wealthy and poor. Not being able to fix depression in our family, especially our children, induce in us a sense of guilt and failure. While we meet depression solely on a personal rather than a professional level, we will always fear the thing we exile, and experience a deep sense of having failed.

Chapter 10

Spiritual Depression

In 2011, I was fortunate to attend the first 'Madness and Literature' at Nottingham University. My particular interest and reason for going was to meet one of the key speakers, American psychiatrist, Kay Redfield Jamison, whose books had been so illuminating and helpful to many. Furthermore, she was one of the main guest speakers.

What I liked about this excellent three-day conference was the sheer diversity of content and openness of the speakers which included Hilary Mantel, author of *Wolf Hall*, Mark Radcliff, author of *Gabriel's Angel* and editor of *The Nursing Times*. I was inspired by the enthusiasm, and knowledge which was brought to bear on such a socially misunderstood subject. Many of the people attending this event were traveling from all over the world, with either personal input of their own struggles or were health professionals working in psychiatry who were able to share input and, more importantly, were able to *receive* input as well.

One of the books on display that drew me was *Spirituality and Psychiatry,* jointly edited by Andrew Sims, former president of the Royal Society of Psychiatrists, Andrew Powell, Senior Lecturer in Psychiatry at St George's Hospital in London, and Chris Cooke, Professional Research Fellow.

I have dipped into this work many times and have been particularly impressed with the chapters on *Neuroscience of the Spirit* and *Spiritual Care in the NHS*, especially as I have worked in this field for 14 years. Within that time, I had observed the paucity of healthcare available to mental health users.

Patients presenting with a health condition with underlying psychiatric symptoms are passed from pillar to post like hot potatoes. Due to ongoing cutbacks in mental health, there are never enough psychiatrists to process each patient's needs. Mental health is certainly the Cinderella of the health profession and, until consciousness changes towards mental health conditions, this will become an ever increasing problem.

As human beings, we are so much more than our physical body and mind. Like the layers of an onion, our consciousness extends into different areas, each with its own viewing lens. As cited in the introduction, these layers are physical, cultural, mental, emotional, psychological and spiritual. Each layer of being is of equal importance, fitting like Nesting Russian Dolls inside each other. Most of the time, we confine our interactive consciousness to the mental, physical and emotional level. Psychological awareness is a skill which develops over time and isn't necessarily a linear process. As children we live more in our emotions which are raw, spontaneous and volatile alongside the dimensions of our physical world. It is only when we have difficult and challenging relationships with others that any self-awareness makes its presence known. In the midst of social conflict emotions will become prominent as the ego finds a way of protecting us from emotional harm by strong defense mechanisms, such as 'denial' and 'splitting'. This is when we cut ourselves off from our feelings because they are too painful to look at. As children, we are held in the family matrix and so our viewing lens into internal and social dynamics will be protected. We will learn which behavior is considered to be acceptable or not. But, outside the family matrix, which doesn't always present an unbiased or clear perspective, other states of consciousness come into operation which may affect our thoughts and feelings.

Perhaps the most dynamic factor which will affect many of us is falling in love. Dynamic, because love animates all the other lenses, it is prismatic and multi-dimensional. As our partner-in-love will, unconsciously, mirror our longings, insecurities and disappointments so their presence becomes larger-than-life.

Personality traits that were repressed emerge through our dreams *and* waking consciousness. Being 'in love' has a way of stirring up the muddy depths of our inner being causing memories that were hidden before to surface. At this critical juncture in the relationship, it takes courage to *stay with* all the feelings and impressions which can be explosive and shatter the image we held of ourselves. Yet, it is important that this point is reached for the relationship to develop onto the next level which is one of commitment. But many young people are not ready for this and, similarly, more mature people who adopt *Peter Pan* roles will scoot off at the first whiff of being tied down and find someone else to enchant.

Yet, in every relationship, something is conceived in the form of a physical child, a creative idea or the opportunity to salvage broken pieces of ourselves through the support of friends, colleagues and, some time later, counseling and therapy. It takes time, energy, financial resources and courage to develop psychological awareness. If we don't feel ready or have a support network strong enough to support us, it may be safer to postpone confronting these areas of the past on a psychological level until we have more stability in our life.

Conversely, the spiritual aspect of our make-up may not become available until we are much older. Alternatively, if we are from a religious background, steeped in these values, we may need to put certain conditions on hold, so that we can develop in ways that are more immediate and accessible to us.

Underlying this, there is a very good reason why anyone wanting to study the mystical 12th-century Judaic Kabbalah were dissuaded from doing this until they had reached a certain degree of psychological maturity. Working in the world of matter with all its disappointments and frustration was held to be a valuable foundation for inner development and maturity. Without personal insight into the everyday world, the young would-be spiritual student does not possess the psychological and emotional maturity to partake of the rigorous lessons until they have reached a greater level of maturity and insight.

Supporting this outlook with scientific data, the prefrontal cortex (PFC) is under-developed in the teenager and does not reach full maturity until they have reached 25 years old. Since the prefrontal cortex controls impulses and strong emotions, this area is important for exercising self-control. Basically, the adolescent's ability to weigh up situations is compromised by the immaturity of their prefrontal cortex. This is because the synapses which connect it to other parts of the brain have not reached developmental maturity. Literally, there are loose wires! Until this connectivity takes place, there is a risk of the young student's emotions being too volatile to undertake such a spiritually disciplined task. In the same context, lowering the voting age from 21 to 18 in the UK seems questionable.

Before going any further, it is important to make a clear distinction between religion and spirituality because they are not always interchangeable. The root word 're-ligion' derives from 'ligaur' which means 'bind to'. Although a religion may harness and evoke an innate sense of spirituality in the individual, they are unique to each other. Religion itself can be dogmatic and define the parameters of a belief system, much like the structure of an unfurnished house. But spirituality is the essence which flows through the rooms, imparting its unique fragrance. But religion on its own is not 'spirituality'. In a sense, many of us have strong views which we feel zealous and religious about. The stronger and more 'binding' our views, the more religious we are. Religion is exoteric, bound to structure and belief. Spirituality is esoteric, the scent of the wind bringing fragrances from afar. Unlike religion which can come into form through ritual, prayer and 'almsgiving', it cannot be bound to form. It is an essence which invokes a sense of awe in us, lifting us out of the mundane. Perhaps I can offer an example of this through the lens of my own experience:

A few months ago, I was taking my whippet for a walk around a nearby wildlife reserve owned by the RSPB. Dusk was beginning to descend, but then we both looked up at the sound of approaching geese overhead. I estimated that there were two or three hundred passing in wave after wave overhead. The sight was awesome, filling me with a sense of wonder and inspiration along with that 'larger than life' feeling that I was connected to a force so much greater than myself; something which was ancient, primeval yet deeply spiritual at the same time. My heart lifted and I felt as though I had been touched by something that is rare and beautiful. There was a longing in me to go with them, to become swept up within their sense of purpose which traversed the mundane.

Experiences like this are timeless and spontaneous. They touch the heart and engage the soul.

In short, it is difficult to get a handle on spirituality. The concept of religion can evoke powerful feelings of devotion, antipathy and guilt. When we communicate about religion, finding our words usually is not much of a problem – unless we become overcome by emotions! Similarly, in any psychotherapeutic relationship, there is a terminology which spills over into everyday language. Words such as *mirroring, wounded, defensemechanisms* and *denial* are descriptive terms which are self-explanatory. But – we do not always have a language for spirituality. We might describe an experience of this nature as 'awesome', 'unifying' or 'out of this world'. But these descriptions can be alienating, further separating us from what is, essentially, a very real experience. In order to get a handle on a spiritual experience we often refer to it as 'religious'. But then we become bound by the word itself. Experience then becomes lost as it becomes imprisoned in form.

Ironically, the more we try to name our experience of spirituality, the more intangible it becomes. The experience, or insight, slips away like blossom or seed fluff in the breeze. This is the distinction between a spiritual and psychic experience. Spirituality is not embedded in our language structure because it is a difficult concept to define. The more we try to bind what is essentially spiritual into language, the more its essence slips away and begins to pale. Yet...

The sacred underpins spiritual experience and what is sacred we, wisely, don't share with 'all and sundry'. In psychological terms a spiritual experience is often described as 'trans-personal' which means beyond the 'self'. The spiritual lends itself well to the creative process in the form of moments of insights – more commonly referred to as the 'ah-ha' experience. Insight happens when everything we have been struggling with comes together in one enlightening moment.

Historically, there are religious and non-religious individuals who have had enlightened experiences which form the direction of their life's work. Usually, this manifests on the heels of a long and protracted period of suffering or struggling on both an inner and outer level. St John of the Cross suffered a long and relentless period of imprisonment yet, simultaneously, experienced an epiphany in the midst of it. Out of this emerged his classic masterpiece, *Dark Night of the Soul*. Here he makes a distinction between *Dark Night of the Senses* and *Dark Night of the Spirit*.

Then, in the Far East, there is the young Prince Siddhartha, the Buddha-to-be who, after being kept ignorant of the suffering in the world by his wealthy parents, slips away on his own to explore what lies beyond the palace for himself. Presently, his journey takes him away from his familiar idyllic home to areas where there is poverty, illness, old age, grief and starvation. Yet... his parents had very good reason for protecting him from the outside world. A seer had once warned them that that their son would become a holy man and leave them one day.

The young Siddhartha's travels took him far and wide on his quest to understand the meaning of suffering. He quickly found that sickness, death and old age were everywhere. There seemed to be nowhere that it was not. Furthermore, he was to discover that even animals were caught up in this endless cycle of suffering too – mainly because of man's relentless cruelty to them. It was for this reason that he chose not to eat meat or wear any product which was made from their flesh or body. After all his traveling and spiritual practice he came to accept that all sentient beings were connected to the 'Wheel of Karma' which was basically an endless process of reincarnation into physical matter through the law of cause and effect. Basically, all selfish and cruel acts which work against the Law of Love create challenging conditions which caution us to atone for our 'sins'. Through each lifetime we have the opportunity to redeem ourselves and work through past karma until we reach enlightenment. This philosophy was to be the driving force which shaped Siddhartha's life journey – to find the meaning of suffering.

To the sadness of his parents who had tried so hard to protect him from the world outside the palace, he left home and thus fulfilled the prophecy the Seer had made before his birth. Meditating for many years in his search for meaning, he was to receive enlightenment and founded the four noble truths upon which Buddhism rests. These are:

Life Means Suffering
The Origin of Suffering is Attachment
The Cessation of Suffering is Attainable
The Path to the Cessation of Suffering

Just as friendship and a social network will confer a sense of belonging and grounding within our environment, connecting with our innate spirituality confers a deep sense of union with all life, both in its smallness and immensity. In this, we experience a greater sense of *purpose, value* and *meaning* in our life. In fact, unless we have these three components in life, we become driven

73

to keep reaching out on a temporal level for our sustenance and, yet find none—or, at least, none that is lasting. Material commodities or even our close friends and relatives cannot address that sense of hunger and longing. In fact, without these values we become emotionally and spiritually impoverished and driven by desperation to escape or distract ourselves from the wolf biting at our heels. While it is true, commodities will make us more comfortable and less anxious; the emotional feedback loop is transitory. An insatiable longing sets in again because no amount of money and worldly distraction can make us happy. This is not to say material resources are wrong in themselves because they are necessary to our health, comfort and contentment. As long as there is a sense of inner value outside, then we are less likely to become dependent on them for our sense of well-being and purpose. Like anything, money can be held lightly.

I am also including here our preoccupation with holidays. For the past few decades it has become possible for most people to travel and take a holiday which can be inspirational and restore one's sense of well-being. But the enjoyment and sense of well-being that a holiday can confer seems to evaporate the moment we return to home ground again. It is this residual hunger which fuels a hunger for the next holiday or next fix.

The interesting thing here is that the root word for 'holiday' has origins in 'holy' and is also related to health. Many of us do take holidays for health reasons, to lessen the stress of living in the Western world. But, before the 12th century, holy days were set aside for worship and spiritual contemplation. The word 'holiday' entered our language halfway through the nineteenth century. So holidays were actually 'holy days' reserved for religious contemplation. I suspect the act of getting away from normal everyday life—the mundane and material is closely connected to making a spiritual pilgrimage.

But let's look at 'spiritual' again which in Latin means

'inspired'. Although there is a growing percentage of people who go on meaningful holidays, there are many who just want to 'let their hair down' and have pleasure. Really, the need for inspiration becomes implemented on a more somatic level rather than an inspirational one. There is a sense of connecting with the 'spirit' in the form of liquor and alcohol. Thus imbibed, it is easy to convince ourselves that we are having a wonderful time. In a sense, 'holy days' have been transformed into spirit-filled ones. Yet... Underlying this is an often unconscious need to become elevated; enlivened by something greater than ourselves. Until this need becomes realized and made conscious, we cannot become spiritually aware. To reach this realization, the longing within us needs to grow in order to eclipse our enjoyment of 'having a good time'. But this is a hard step to negotiate because consciousness is both threatening and life-changing. Reaching rock bottom may be the only step available. It is often this sense of emptiness and growing awareness of what is missing which drives us into a state of depression.

In the next chapter, I want to explore the relationship between alcoholism and depression.

Chapter 11

Alcoholism and Depression

Alcoholism and depression have an intimate connection with each other.

Swiss Psychiatrist, Carl Jung, and Bill Wilson, the founder of Alcoholics Anonymous (AA), were in communication on several occasions over the relationship between alcoholism and depression. Together, they agreed that alcoholism was often a substitute for lack of faith in a 'Higher Power', or a spiritual anchor.

An interesting point to add here is that Bill Wilson suffered from depression himself as had his Grandfather. Primarily, all Bill's attempts to give up alcohol came to nothing until, in desperation, he prayed for the strength to give up alcohol as he knew he couldn't do this on his own. Soon after this he became aware of a bright light, a feeling of ecstasy and a great peace and his prayer was soon answered. This is where his belief in a Higher Power came in and was to become the 2nd step of the AA program: *We came to believe that a Power greater than ourselves can deliver us to sanity.*

Yet, before this second step could be taken the alcoholic has to realize and adhere to the first step: *We admitted we were powerless over alcohol and that our lives had become unmanageable.*

Realizing the strength of this *power*, Wilson wanted to make this an important component of the recovery program. He believed that the form the Higher Power presented itself in was unique to each individual, whatever religion they followed. In the context of this chapter, the unnamed power was a spiritual one. This spirituality came into form through the AA network worldwide.

It is ironic that people resort to alcohol in an effort to mitigate feelings of anxiety, nervousness and low self-worth which, when it has run its short-lived course, leaves them with depression and all the symptoms that caused them to drink in the first place. The ebullience which alcohol offered a few hours previously, gives way to the very feelings that they tried so hard to escape from.

I have to say, that for the average person who doesn't have an addictive personality, it is not usually a problem. Because the *average person* can stop at one drink or even have too many sometimes, and not become reliant on it.

Yet, the majority of alcoholics haven't chosen to be that way. Many people who suffer from depression self-medicate to alleviate and forget about their pain. It is common knowledge that a third of all substance abusers suffer from depression. As depression has strong hereditary factors, so does alcoholism and this is why they are so closely linked.

Next I want to look at the value of the Black Dog.

Chapter 12

The Value of the Black Dog

Because value is not something which, in our western culture, is equated with depression, it is hard to understand its connection to such a debilitating condition. How can a disease that diminishes self-esteem, sabotages the very fabric of one's life, crucifies the body, tortures the mind, silences the emotions, exiles the spirit, have any value? Isn't this like believing in miracles? Or turning stones into bread? Or the alchemy of base metals into gold?

In this context, I am thinking of the linear way we perceive any life experience, where everything is sorted into two boxes, one marked 'bad' the other 'good'. Like a black-and-white chessboard we only want to remain on the white squares. What is known and understood is safer and preferable. But then, if there was no darkness, the white squares would not show up any more than the stars in the nighttime sky. These extremes are everywhere and are part of the duality we are familiar with. Weaned on the idyllic vision of the good overcoming bad, we become filled with shame and anger when this is not always so in our own lives. Yet, each day, we walk step-by-step with duality; whether this is bearing witness to the day passing into night and vice versa, or fall tipping into winter—becoming spring and then summer. In one country, people are enjoying abundance in food and water. Yet in another part of the world there is poverty and malnutrition. Globally, there are areas of verdant rain forest, in another aridity and still others with oceans and rivers forming connections across the world. In another, there is kilometer upon kilometer of desert where water and food is scarce. Although extremes are more pronounced today with global weather changes, deforestation and pollution there have always been extreme polarities in climate, light and darkness. These polarities underpin the flow of migration from the Arctic terns to the caribou and Monarch butterfly. In the winter we long for the first bud, the growing warmth and lushness of the earth as its multi-colored robe embroiders the landscape.

Yet, when we apply this same model to ourselves, why does one polarity hold more value than the other? Here, we come up against a powerful cultural lens which is focused on achievement, prosperity, productivity, health and happiness. Anything other than being rich, successful and healthy falls short of this impossible template of perfection and achievement.

This artificially manufactured lens creates a 'no-win' situation whereby, investment in this belief, will always cause us to fall short. We have failed by our humanness. Yet, each day, we are challenged to come home to our true self by daring to embrace the 'dark' side within nature and ourselves.

Let us not forget that depression is *big* business, as are all the other aberrations listed in the Diagnostic Manual of Mental Health, whose umbrella of ailments, real or imagined, expand at such a rate that it is running ahead of itself like a shadow escaping the sun. Now that this is all out in the open, the messiness and greed of the predatory forces that are targeting every ailment in the form of modern medicine invites the question – where do we go from here?

We stay still. Own our differences which hold the seeds of genius and invention which, like Brighton candy rock duplicates itself through every century, each new generation. If depression hadn't been around, maybe Newton would never have invented gravity or John Ruskin written his luminous works on nature, or Gerald Manley Hopkins and Sylvia Plath and so many others written their iconic poetry. In short, without these so-called flaws in individual make-up, the world would lose much of its poetry, music and words. For these so-called 'flaws' of temperament keep us culturally rich.

Forget about shooting, beating, whipping the Black Dog. The Black Dog has been around for centuries and shows very little sign of going away. Tethered to an ever growing roll call of antidepressant and antipsychotic medication, it keeps us afraid, exasperated, defensive, yet strangely fascinated by its tenacity, power and resilience. Furthermore, it has a real message which runs counter to our current mindset: that depression has no value.

The message is this: it *does* have value and anything of value is always threatened and undermined. That is like saying that if life is challenging and difficult, even unbearable at times, it has no value. Rather than fixating on the deficits—what it takes away in the form of happiness, hope and trust, I want to focus on the qualities which depression confers instead; qualities which psychiatrists such as Peter Kramer, Thomas Moore, Kay Redfield Jamieson and Martha Manning describe throughout their writing in the form of creativity and wisdom, although on a monetary level, one cannot put a price on these.

Again, I have to say that in a world which is enthralled by success, money, happiness there is very little chance or opportunity to harness the *value* of dis-ease and depression. Nelson Mandela didn't develop peace of mind, wisdom and insight overnight. Before he was imprisoned for 27 years he was a headstrong and impatient young man. Yet, finally on his release, he admitted, he was neither broken nor defeated.

Somewhere in the midst of his grueling imprisonment he found the tools to fashion a whole new way of looking at life along with an unwavering vision for the future.

I list some of these qualities emerging through depression here:

Resilience
Strength
Staying power

Empathy
Insight
Determination
Creativity

These are no mean qualities. Although we may be born with the potential to develop these qualities through genetic inheritance and sheer willpower, most of the time they develop through trial-and-error together with a vast amount of self-discipline. Without resilience, strength and staying power the task cannot be completed as is evident in someone who has the initial will to start a project, but not the staying power to complete it. Without this there is a tendency to leave behind a battalion of half-completed projects. The will may be there in the beginning, but can quickly peter out, leaving behind a trail of half-finished projects.

Yet because of the sense of being locked in a silent battle with a depressive condition, strength, resilience and staying power have the opportunity to come to the fore. I have heard it said that creativity, in whatever form it manifests, is one percent inspiration and 99% hard work. Certainly, I have found this to be true for myself.

Actually, inspiration is the easy part and is free. It is available to everyone if they want to take it on. It just wafts in like seed fluff, ready to lodge with us if we dare to make the commitment or allow this visitor our time. But, in order to keep that seed fluff, we have to grasp it there and then. The seeds of inspiration are wandersome and elusive. The moment we reach out to grab them, they waft away in search of another home to lodge in. And although we are visited by these seeded parachutes daily in the form of inspiration or a calling, we dismiss them as having no value because they are *free* and, therefore, worthless. If they were priceless as inherently they are, we would be fighting over them!

The quality of empathy is not only available to those suffering with depression, but there for anyone who struggles on a daily basis with any level of suffering. Bitterness and anger may close the door to this. But if these emotions eclipse the heart for too long, empathy may never have the chance to develop. Bitterness and anger are not our natural state of being, although they have their purpose. Especially anger, as this energizes us to move forward and resolve the trauma which is holding us back. In contrast, bitterness can erode our will to move forward and hold us hostage so that we lack the energy to move onto new ground.

But the real strength to move forward is in the surrendering, the acceptance and the letting go.

Bibliography

Agahdiu, Mabel. *Soul Matters: the spiritual dimension within healthcare*, Radcliffe Publishing, 2010

Assagioli, Roberto. *Psychosynthesis*, HarperCollins, 1993

Cantopher, Tim. *Depressive illness: The Curse of the Strong*, Sheldon Press, Third Edition, 2012

Kramer, Peter. *Against Depression*, Penguin Group, USA, 2005

Jamison Redfield, Kay. *Touched with Fire: Manic-Depressive Illness and the Artistic Temperament*, Free Press Paperbacks, 1996

Sorrell, Stephanie. *Depression as a Spiritual Journey*, Psyche Books, 2009

Rosenthal, Norman. *Winter Blues*, The Guildford Press, 2012 (Fourth Edition)

Karp, David. *Speaking of Sadness*, Oxford University Press, 1996

Frankl, Victor. *Man's Search for Meaning*, Beacon Press, 2006

Manning, Martha. *Undercurrents*, HarperCollins, 1994

Ghaemi, Nassir. *A First-Rate Madness*, Penguin Group, 2011

Oxley-Rice, Mark. *Underneath the Lemon Tree*, Little Brown, 2012

Shenk, Joshua Wolf. *Lincoln's Melancholy*, Boston: Houghton Mifflin, 2005

Solomon, Andrew. *The Noonday Demon*, Chatto & Windus, 2001

Starr, Mirabai. *Dark Night of the Soul*, Riverhead Books, 2002

Recommended Reading
Cook, Chris. (ed), Powell, Andrew and Sims, Andrew. *Spirituality and psychiatry*, Royal College of Psychiatrists, 2009

**PSYCHE
BOOKS**

The study of the mind: interactions, behaviours, functions.
Developing and learning our understanding of self. Psyche
Books cover all aspects of psychology and matters relating to
the head.